JUICING FOR A VIBRANT AND HEALTHFUL EXISTENCE

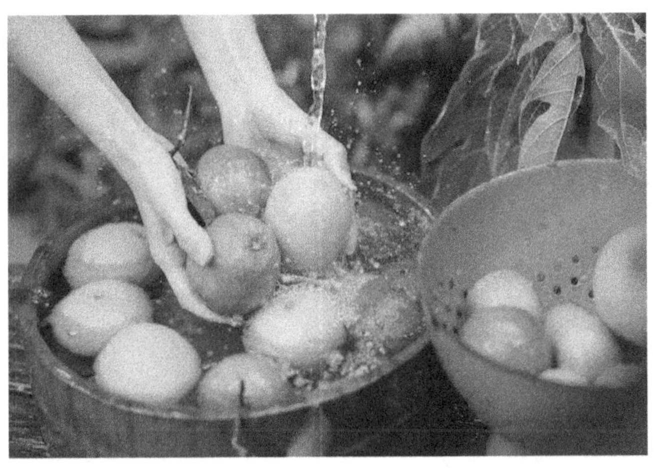

A book on the positive impact of juicing

Kimberly Cline

Table of Contents

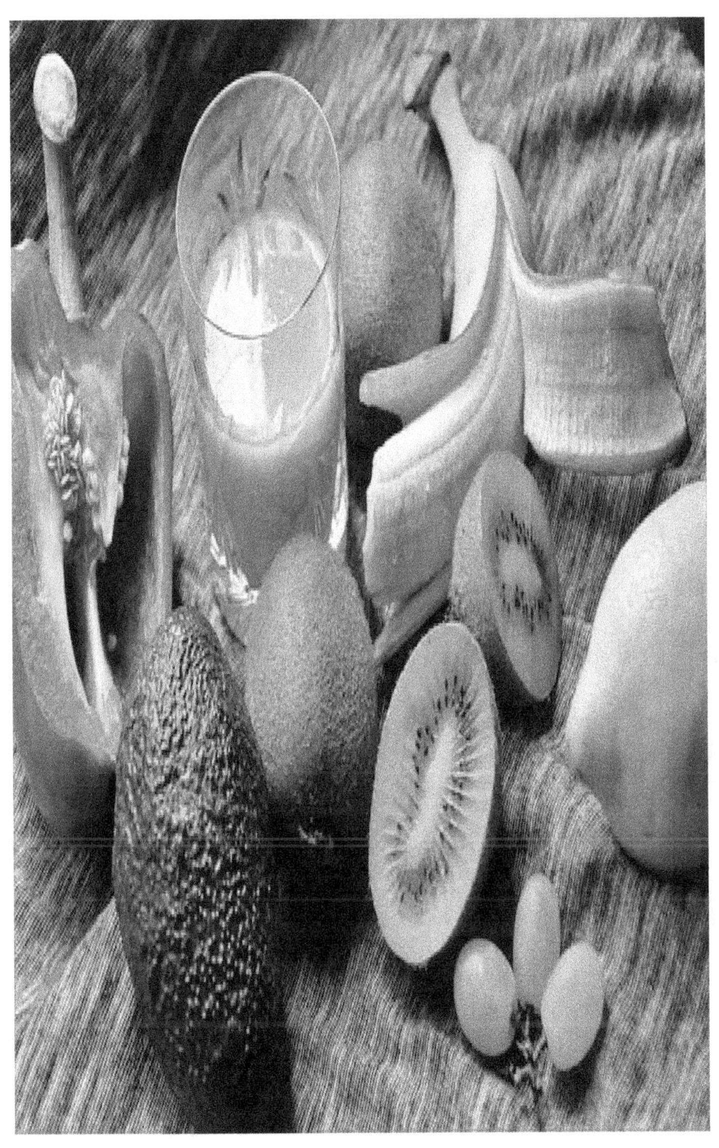

Introduction

Sarah had always struggled with her health. She longed for a vibrant lifestyle, free from lethargy and defeat. One day, she stumbled upon a juicing book that promised a rejuvenating path to wellness. Curiosity grabbed hold, and Sarah immersed herself in its pages, learning about the myriad of fruits and vegetables that could transform her life. Inspired and determined, she purchased a juicer and began her journey to radiant health. Each morning, she would wake up excitedly, concocting vibrant blends that nourished her body and uplifted her spirit. Through the juicing book, Sarah found her path to a healthful life, filling her days with energy and joy.

In a world where fast food and processed snacks dominate, it's becoming more important than ever to prioritize our health and well-being. If you're looking to make a positive change in your life, then juicing might just be the answer you've been searching for.

Introducing "Juicing for a Vibrant and Healthful Existence," a book packed with all the information, and tips you need to embark on an incredible journey towards a healthier, more vibrant life.

This captivating guide is designed to inspire and empower you, teaching you the wonders of juicing and how it can transform your mind, body, and spirit. Discover the incredible health benefits of fresh, nutrient-dense juices and learn how they can help fight off diseases, boost your immune system, and enhance your overall well-being.

But juicing isn't just about the physical benefits – it's also a gateway to a whole new world of flavors and tastes. So, if you're ready to take control of your health and embark on a journey towards a more vibrant and healthful existence, then "Juicing for a Vibrant and Healthful Existence" is for you.

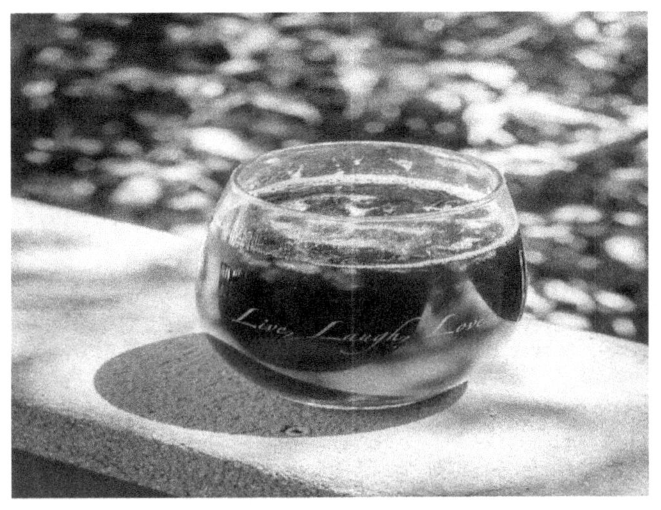

Live, Laugh, Love

Chapter 1: Introduction to Juicing

With more people attempting to enhance their health and well-being, juicing has grown in popularity over time. Juice from fruits and vegetables is extracted in this process, offering a concentrated dose of nutrients and antioxidants. Juicing is an easy way to incorporate a variety of fruits and vegetables into your diet and can be a convenient way to consume your daily recommended intake. Many people enjoy the vibrant flavors and vibrant colors that juices offer, making them an enjoyable and refreshing addition to their routine.

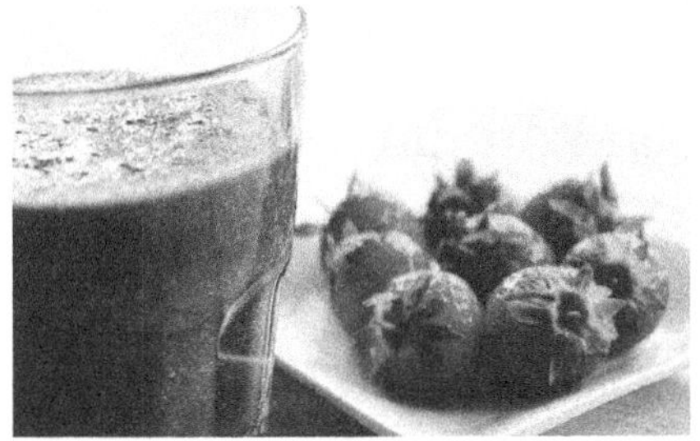

Definition and Benefits of Juicing

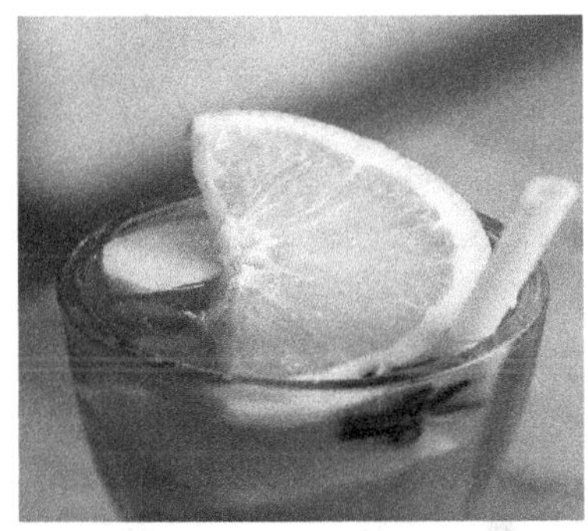

Juicing refers to the process of extracting juice from fruits and vegetables to create a nutrient-packed drink. It allows for quick absorption of vitamins, minerals, and antioxidants. Consuming freshly made juice can boost immunity, improve digestion, detoxify the body, and promote weight loss. It also provides a convenient way to increase fruit and vegetable intake, especially for those who have difficulty consuming them in their whole form. Additionally, juicing can improve skin health, boost energy levels, and support overall well-being.

History and Origin of Juicing

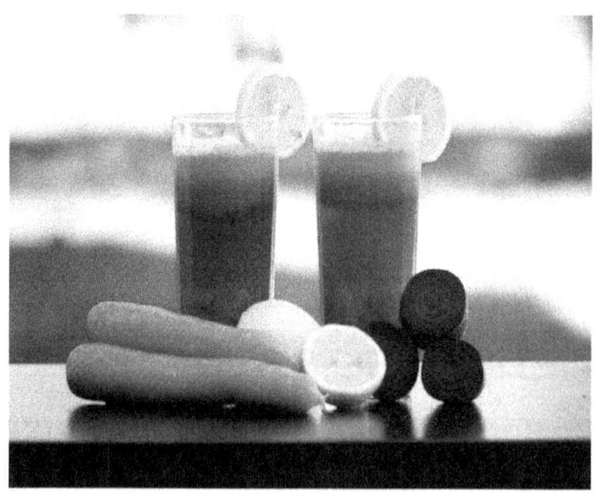

Juicing is not a new concept, as it dates back thousands of years to ancient civilizations. The history and origin of juicing can be traced to the use of various plants and fruits in traditional medicines. The Egyptians were known to extract juices from plants for medicinal purposes, while the Romans and Greeks also used juices as health tonics. Over time, juicing has evolved, and today it is popularized as a convenient and efficient way to consume essential nutrients and improve overall health.

Exploring the Different Types of Juicers and Their Functionalities

Juicing has gained popularity as a trend in health care and for a good cause. Juices that have just been prepared are bursting with vitamins, minerals, and enzymes that can improve our general health. However, choosing the best juicer might be overwhelming given the abundance of options available. Centrifugal and masticating juicers are the two most prevalent varieties. Using a fast-spinning blade, centrifugal juicers extract juice from fruits and vegetables. They are quick and convenient but may not be as efficient at extracting all the nutrients. On the other hand, masticating juicers crush the ingredients slowly to extract the juice. This method preserves more nutrients and allows for a higher juice yield. They are also suitable for juicing leafy greens and wheatgrass. Ultimately, the best juicer for you will depend on your personal preferences and juicing needs.

Understanding the Difference Between Juice and Smoothies

Juice and smoothies are both popular options for consuming fruits and vegetables, but they have key differences. Juice is made by extracting the liquid from fruits and vegetables, removing the fiber. This results in a concentrated source of vitamins and minerals, but without the filling fiber. Smoothies, on the other hand, are made by blending whole fruits and vegetables, including fiber. This provides a more balanced and filling option, with a slower release of nutrients. Choose the option that best suits your needs and dietary preferences.

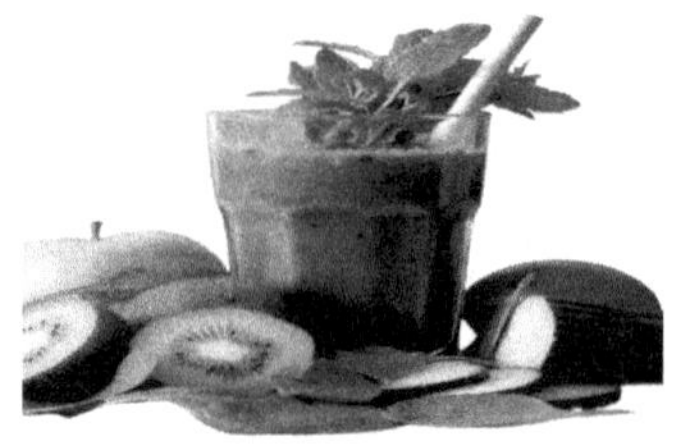

Tips for Selecting and Storing Fresh Produce for Juicing

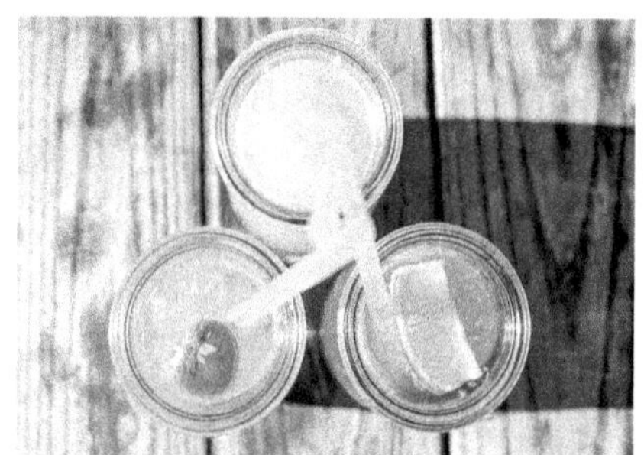

When it comes to juicing, it's important to select and store fresh produce properly to ensure the best flavor and nutritional value. Look for fruits and vegetables that are firm, free of bruises or blemishes, and have vibrant colors. When feasible, choose organic produce to prevent exposure to dangerous pesticides. Store your fruits and vegetables in the refrigerator to keep them fresh and retain their nutrients. Avoid storing produce near fruits that produce ethylene gas, as it can cause premature ripening and spoilage.

Safety Precautions to Keep in Mind While Juicing

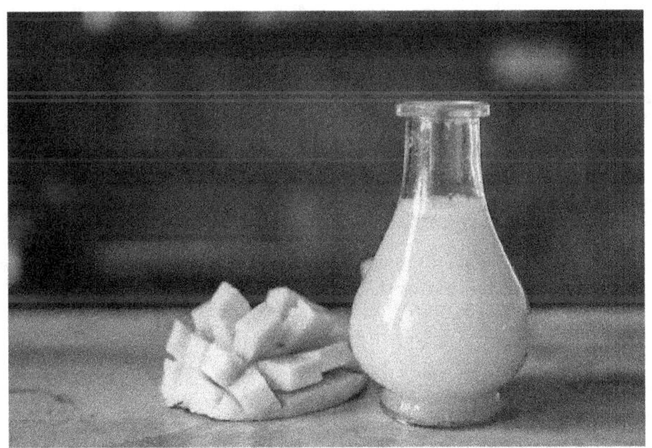

Juicing is a popular way to incorporate fruits and vegetables into our diets, but it's important to prioritize safety while using a juicer. First, ensure that your juicer is clean and properly disinfected before each use. Use only fresh produce and wash them thoroughly to remove any dirt, pesticides, or bacteria. Additionally, be cautious with your fingers and use the pusher to feed produce into the juicer to avoid any accidents. Finally, follow the manufacturer's instructions and guidelines to prevent any mishaps and enjoy your fresh juice with peace of mind.

Understanding Nutritional Needs

Understanding nutritional needs while juicing is essential to ensure that you are getting the right balance of vitamins, minerals, and nutrients. It is important to include a variety of fruits, vegetables, and other ingredients to ensure that you are getting a wide range of nutrients. Additionally, to meet your specific nutritional needs, it may be necessary to supplement certain nutrients or consult with a nutritionist or dietitian for guidance.

The Significance of Comprehending Individual Dietary Requirements

Understanding individual dietary requirements is crucial when it comes to juicing. Because everyone has different dietary requirements, what works for one person might not be suitable for another. By comprehending individual dietary requirements, you can tailor your juicing recipes to meet specific needs, such as increasing nutrient intake, supporting weight loss, or managing chronic health conditions. Additionally, understanding dietary requirements can help prevent harmful interactions between medications and certain ingredients in the juice. Overall, considering individual dietary requirements while juicing ensures that the juice is both safe and effective for the individual's specific needs.

Chapter 2: Exploring Essential Vitamins and Minerals Found in Fruits and Vegetables

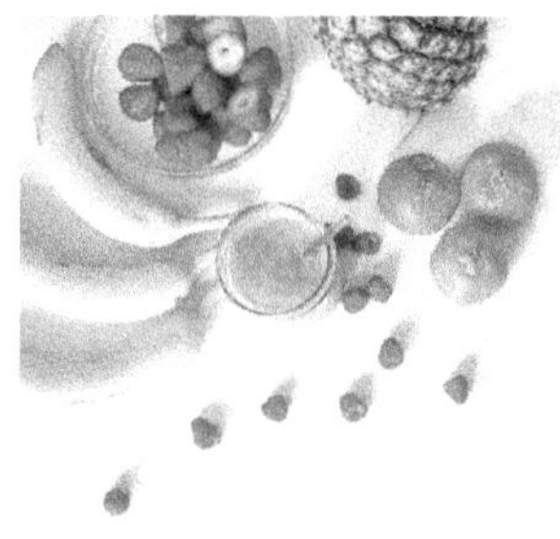

Fruits and vegetables are rich in essential vitamins and minerals that are vital for our overall health. They provide us with a wide range of nutrients, including vitamin C, vitamin A, potassium, magnesium, and calcium. These nutrients play a crucial role in maintaining proper immune function, promoting healthy skin, supporting strong bones, and aiding digestion. Incorporating a variety of fruits and vegetables into our diet ensures we receive the necessary vitamins and minerals our body needs.

How Juicing Can Help Fulfill Daily Nutritional Requirements

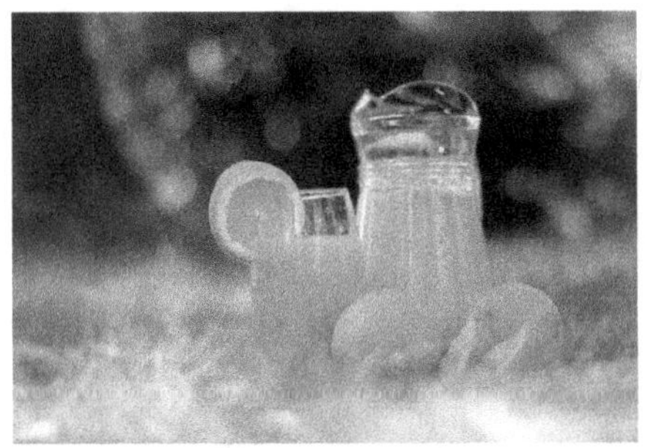

Juicing is a popular way to increase nutrient intake and meet daily nutritional requirements. Freshly squeezed fruits and vegetables are packed with vitamins, minerals, and antioxidants that support overall health. Juicing allows for quick absorption, providing a concentrated dose of essential nutrients that can boost energy levels and promote well-being.

The Role of Various Fruits and Vegetables in Promoting Overall Health and Vitality

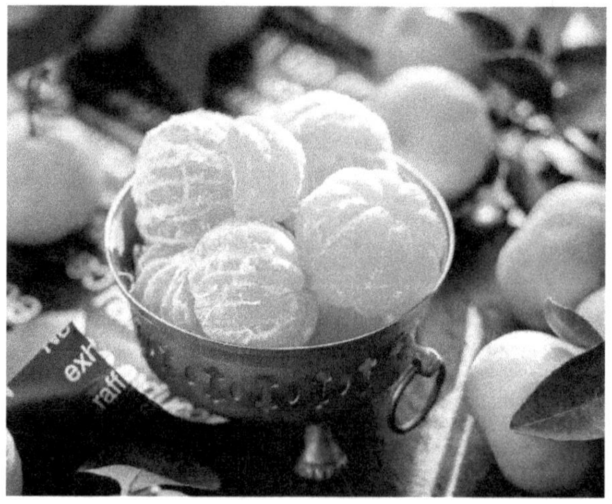

Eating a variety of fruits and vegetables is essential for maintaining overall health and vitality. Each fruit and vegetable offers a unique combination of vitamins, minerals, and antioxidants that contribute to a robust immune system and improved energy levels. For example, citrus fruits like oranges and grapefruits are rich in vitamin C, which boosts the immune system and protects against disease. Leafy green vegetables such as spinach and broccoli are packed with essential nutrients like iron and fiber, crucial for maintaining a healthy digestive system and preventing constipation. Berries, like blueberries and strawberries, are a powerhouse of antioxidants that help to combat free radicals and reduce the risk of chronic diseases, such as cancer and heart disease. Overall, the variety of fruits and vegetables available ensures that we receive a balanced and diverse range of nutrients, promoting overall health and vitality.

Incorporating Juicing Into a Healthy Lifestyle

Incorporating juicing into a healthy lifestyle can provide numerous benefits. Juicing allows you to consume a variety of fruits and vegetables in one drink, providing an abundance of vitamins and minerals. It is also a great way to detoxify the body and boost the immune system.

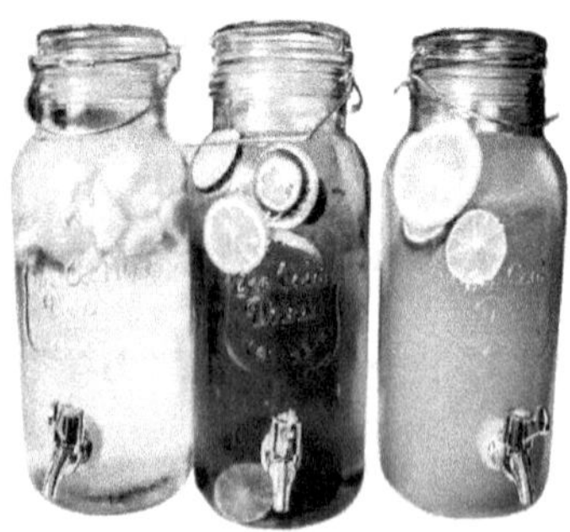

Strategies for Incorporating Juicing Into a Well-balanced Diet

Incorporating juicing into a well-balanced diet can be a great way to increase your intake of fruits and vegetables. One strategy is to start your day with fresh juice made from a variety of produce. Another approach is to replace a snack or meal with a nutrient-rich juice. Additionally, you can use juicing as a way to supplement your regular meals, by adding small amounts of juice to dishes like soups or sauces. It's crucial to keep in mind that juicing shouldn't take the place of eating full fruits and vegetables.

The Role of Juicing in Detoxification and Cleansing

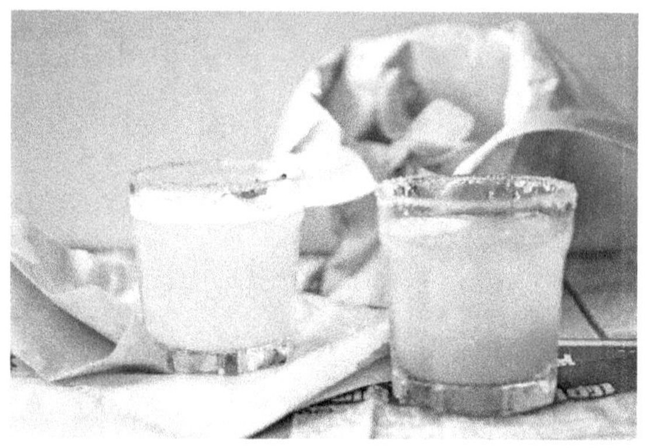

Juicing has gained popularity as a means to detoxify and cleanse the body. By consuming fresh, nutrient-rich juices, individuals can flood their systems with vitamins, minerals, and antioxidants, while giving their digestive system a break from processing solid foods. Juicing also allows the body to easily absorb nutrients, aiding in the elimination of toxins. However, it is important to remember that juicing should be done in moderation and alongside a balanced diet for optimal health benefits.

Tips for Supplementing Juicing With Exercise and Mindfulness Practices

When supplementing juicing with exercise and mindfulness practices, it's important to have a balanced approach. Start by incorporating gentle forms of exercise like yoga or walking while juicing. As your energy levels rise, gradually up the intensity. Mindfulness practices, such as meditation or deep breathing, can enhance your overall well-being. Take the time to understand your body's needs and listen to them.

Remember, rest and recovery are just as important as exercise, so don't forget to schedule some downtime to relax and rejuvenate.

Recipes and Juicing Techniques

Recipes and juicing techniques are a great way to incorporate more fruits and vegetables into your diet. Whether you're looking to boost your immune system, detoxify your body, or simply add more nutrients to your meals, there are endless options to choose from. From green smoothies to vibrant fruit juices, these recipes and techniques will leave you feeling energized and revitalized. Start exploring the world of juicing today!

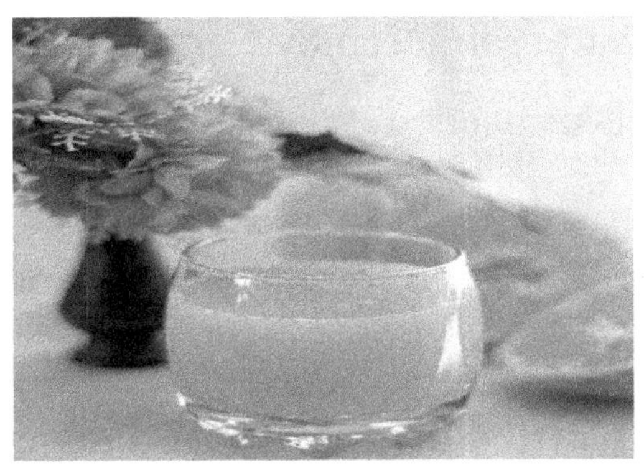

A Step-by-step Guide on Juicing Different Types of Produce

Step 1: Choose your product. Select a variety of fruits and vegetables that you enjoy and that are in season. Some popular choices include apples, oranges, carrots, spinach, and beets.

Step 2: Wash and prepare the produce. Rinse all of the ingredients thoroughly under cool water and remove any stems, leaves, or peels as needed.

Step 3: Cut the produce into small pieces. Your juicer will be able to extract the juice more easily as a result.

Juice the product in step four: Follow the instructions provided by your specific juicer model to extract the juice from each ingredient.

Step 5: Mix and enjoy. Combine the different juices in a glass or container and stir well. Serve your freshly produced juice right away and enjoy!

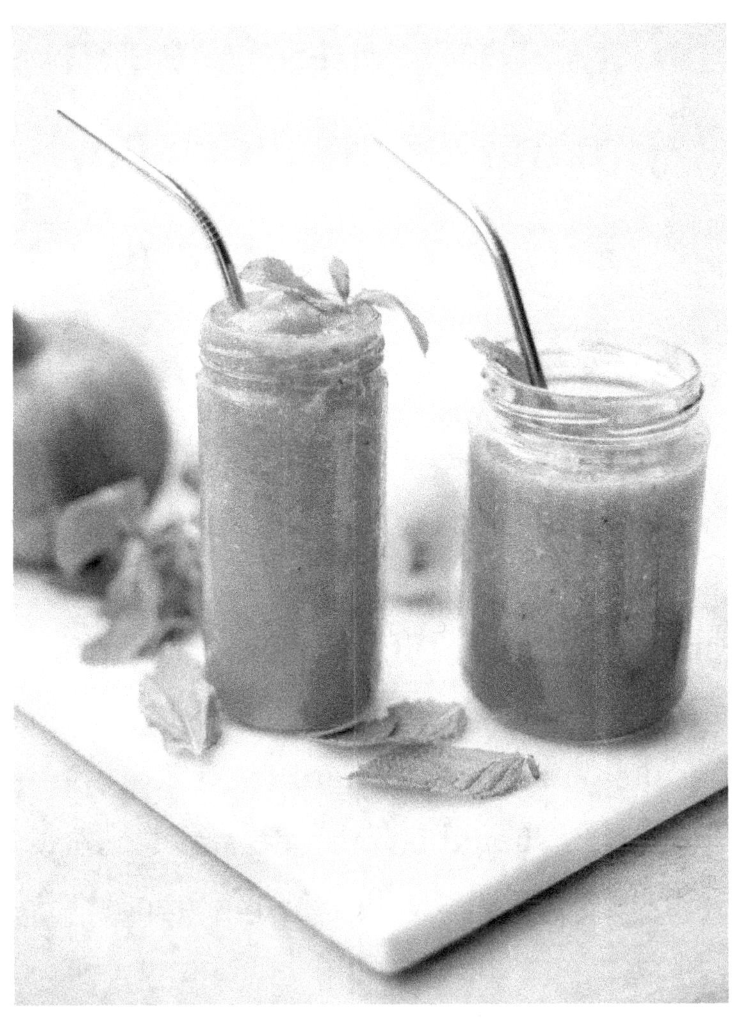

Chapter 3:Variations in Juicing Techniques For Different Fruits and Vegetables

Fruits and vegetables can now be conveniently consumed by juicing. But when it comes to juicing, not all fruits and veggies are made equal. Different products require different juicing techniques to yield the best results. For example, hard fruits like apples and pears should be cut into smaller pieces before juicing, while leafy greens like spinach and kale should be tightly packed and pushed through slowly. Citrus fruits should be peeled before juicing, while soft fruits like berries can be juiced with their seeds intact. By understanding these variations in juicing techniques, you can get the most out of your fruits and vegetables.

Creating Delicious and Nutritious Juice Combinations For Specific Health Goals (e.g., immunity, digestion, and energy)

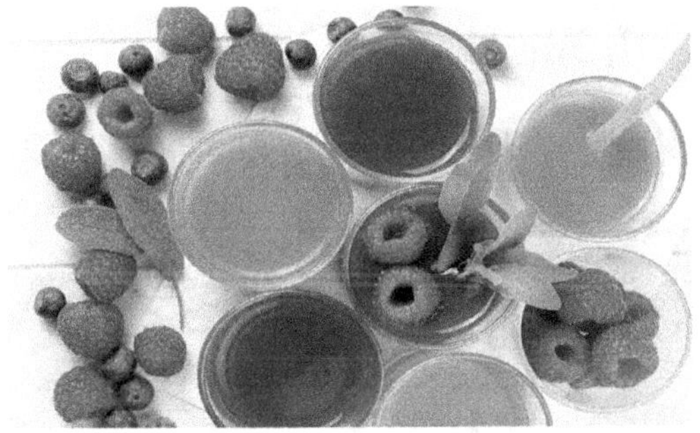

Creating delicious and nutritious juice combinations for specific health goals is a fantastic way to add a boost to your overall well-being. For those aiming to improve their immunity, a combination of citrus fruits like oranges, lemons, and grapefruits can be a great choice due to their high vitamin C content. For better digestion, including ingredients like ginger, pineapple, and papaya can aid in reducing inflammation and improving gut health. If you need an energy boost, a mix of fruits like apples, bananas, and berries can provide natural sugars and antioxidants to keep you energized throughout the day. Experimenting with different combinations can help you discover the perfect juice to meet your specific health goals.

Tips For Proper Juicing Ratios and Ingredient Selection

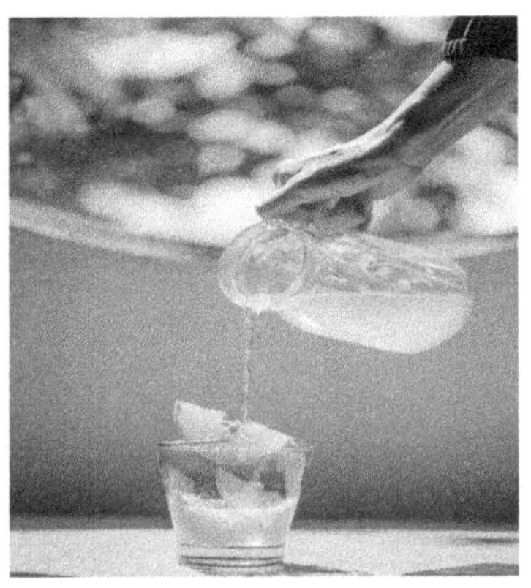

When it comes to juicing, getting the right ratios and ingredient selection is key to achieving the perfect blend of flavors and nutrients. One tip for proper juicing ratios is to balance the sweetness with the acidity. For example, if you're using sweet fruits like apples or oranges, adding a bit of lemon or lime juice can help to cut through the sweetness. Another tip is to experiment with different combinations of fruits and vegetables to create unique flavor profiles. Don't be afraid to mix in some leafy greens like spinach or kale to add a boost of nutrients. Lastly, always make sure to use fresh, organic produce for the best quality juice.

Juicing For Specific Dietary Needs (e.g., vegan, gluten-free)

Juicing is a versatile way to meet specific dietary needs, including vegan and gluten-free diets. For vegans, juicing provides a convenient way to increase the intake of essential nutrients like iron, calcium, and vitamin B12 from plant-based sources. Green juices made from leafy greens, cucumber, and avocado are great options. For those following a gluten-free diet, juicing is a fantastic way to incorporate nutrient-dense fruits and vegetables without any worry of gluten contamination. Be creative, try juicing combinations like beet, carrot, and apple for a refreshing and gluten-free beverage that nourishes your body.

Understanding How Juicing Can Support Specific Health Conditions (e.g., diabetes and high blood pressure)

Juicing has become popular for improving overall health, but it can also be beneficial for managing specific health conditions like diabetes and high blood pressure. Juicing allows for an easy way to consume nutrient-dense foods while being mindful of sugar content for those with diabetes. Green juices with leafy greens, cucumber, and lemon can help regulate blood sugar levels. In the case of high blood pressure, juicing recipes that are high in potassium and nitrates, such as beet, celery, and spinach juice, can support healthy blood flow and lower blood pressure. However, before making any dietary adjustments, it's crucial to speak with a medical expert.

The Importance of Consulting With a Healthcare Professional When Using Juicing as a Complementary Therapy

When considering juicing as a complementary therapy, it is important to consult with a healthcare professional before starting. They can assess your health conditions, help manage potential side effects, and ensure that juicing is safe and beneficial for your individual needs.

Beyond Juicing – Incorporating Juiced Ingredients Into Everyday Life

Beyond Juicing is a fantastic way to bring the benefits of juiced ingredients into your everyday life. Instead of just drinking your favorite fruits and vegetables, why not incorporate them into your meals? Add juiced ingredients to your salads, stir-fries, and sauces for a flavorful and nutritious boost. You can also use juiced ingredients in baking, adding natural sweetness and moisture to your treats. Don't limit yourself to just drinking juice - explore the endless possibilities of Beyond Juicing!

Exploring Ways to Incorporate Juiced Ingredients Into Everyday Recipes (e.g., soups, dressings, smoothies)

Incorporating juiced ingredients into everyday recipes can be a great way to add flavor, nutrition, and variety to your meals. To help you start, here are some suggestions you can consider using as a starting point:

Soups: Use freshly squeezed vegetable or fruit juice as a broth base for soups. For example, you can make a refreshing gazpacho by blending tomato juice with cucumber and bell pepper juice.

Dressings: Replace vinegar or citrus juice in your dressings with freshly squeezed fruit juice. This can add a vibrant and tangy flavor to your salads. Try combining orange juice with olive oil, honey, and Dijon mustard for a citrusy dressing.

Smoothies: Incorporate fresh juice into your smoothies for an extra nutrient boost. For example, add carrot or beet juice to a fruit smoothie for added sweetness and vibrant color.

Marinades: Replace some of the liquid in your marinades with freshly squeezed juice. This can add acidity and flavor to meats and vegetables. For instance, mix lemon juice with garlic, olive oil, and herbs for a refreshing chicken marinade.

Remember to balance the flavors and adjust the quantities of other ingredients to complement the juiced ingredient. Try out various combinations to make delectable and wholesome meals.

Creating a Sustainable Juicing Routine by Minimizing Waste

Creating a sustainable juicing routine involves minimizing waste by making smart choices throughout the process. This can include planning your juicing recipes to use up all parts of the fruits and vegetables, such as the peels and pulp. Additionally, consider composting leftover scraps instead of throwing them away. Using reusable or compostable containers for storage and composting or recycling packaging materials are also important steps in reducing waste and creating a sustainable juicing routine.

Conclusion

In conclusion, juicing offers a multitude of benefits for achieving and maintaining a vibrant and healthful existence. By incorporating fresh, nutrient-rich juices into your daily routine, you can boost your intake of vitamins, minerals, and antioxidants, helping to strengthen your immune system, improve digestion, and promote overall well-being.

Juicing provides a convenient and efficient way to consume a wide variety of fruits and vegetables, ensuring that you receive a diverse range of essential nutrients that may be lacking from your regular diet. These nutrients can help to support healthy bodily functions, strengthen bones and muscles, and protect against chronic diseases.

Moreover, juicing allows for easy absorption and digestion of nutrients, as the juicing process breaks down the cell walls of fruits and vegetables, making the nutrients readily available for your body to absorb. This could assist boost vitality and energy levels all around.

Additionally, the vibrant colors and flavors of fresh juices can make healthy living enjoyable and exciting. Experimenting with different combinations of fruits, vegetables, and herbs can introduce you to new taste sensations and make every juicing experience unique.

Juicing should not take the place of full fruits and vegetables in your diet, it is crucial to remember this. Whole fruits and vegetables contain additional fiber that is crucial for maintaining a healthy digestive system. Therefore, it is best to complement juicing with a balanced diet that includes whole foods.

In conclusion, incorporating juicing into your lifestyle can contribute to a vibrant and healthful existence. It offers a convenient way to increase your intake of essential nutrients, supports a strong immune system, and enhances overall well-being. However, it is important to remember that juicing should be a supplement to, and not a replacement for, whole fruits and vegetables. So go ahead and invest in a good quality juicer, experiment with different combinations, and reap the benefits of a vibrant and healthy life. Cheers to juicing!

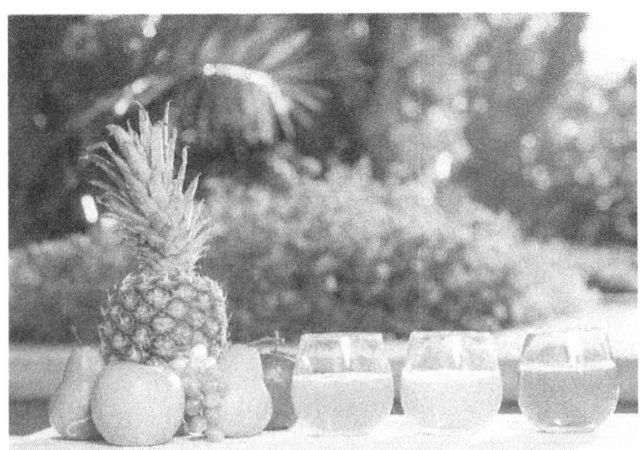